SEXUAL SATISFACTION IN MARRIAGE

KEYS TO SEXUAL SATISFACTION TO SAVE YOUR MARRIAGE

BY

MATHEW J. ASHTON

TABLE OF CONTENTS

INTRODUCTION

SECTION1: UNDERSTAND THE SEXUAL DIFFERENCES BETWEEN MEN AND WOMEN

SECTION2: ELIMINATE THE COMMON ENEMIES OF SEXUAL FULFILLMENT

SECTION3:OVERCOME THE BARRIERS TO FULFILLING SEX

SECTION 4: WORK TO CREATE AN ATMOSPHERE OF SEXUAL PLEASURE

SECTION 5: DO YOUR PART TO KEEP THE ROMANCE ALIVE

CONCLUSION

INTRODUCTION

Like virtually nothing else, sex draws our attention, and for good reason one it's of life's greatest joys. It is also necessary for living a happy life. We feel our best emotionally, psychologically, and physically when we have wonderful sex lives.

Sexual desire is one of the most fundamental and potent human urges, ranking right up there with hunger and thirst, yet it goes well beyond simply serving as a mechanism for species reproduction. Sex is a celebration of a happy existence, a way to connect with a chosen partner, and an expression of perfection. But for far too many couples, the pressures of daily life, aging, or deteriorating health stand in the way of a fulfilling sexual relationship.

This book can assist you in getting back in touch with your sexual energy if you're one of the millions of people who find their Usesexual life to be lacking.

If you are reading this book, it's possible that your long-term, committed relationship has lost some of its spark. You and your partner likely only needed to exchange glances in the beginning across a busy room to set off a series of events that culminated in sexual fireworks. Yet as the years went by, obstacles like children, careers, and normal body wear and tear arose. You might think that getting things going in the bedroom these days requires nothing less than a nuclear reaction. You might believe that this is how things always work out, but it's not. Passionate sex can be present in your now and future as well as only a pleasant recollection from your past.

This tutorial will teach you about the lengthy and fascinating history of food as a source of sexual satisfaction.

SECTION 1

UNDERSTAND THE SEXUAL DIFFERENCES BETWEEN MEN AND WOMEN

We think that having sex is a lovely, divinely-given urge that can unite a husband and wife. We also think that having or not having sex is a good indicator of how committed and intimate you two are to one another in other parts of your marriage. Each partner must take the risk of being completely open and vulnerable to the other for sex to be truly pleasurable for both parties.

Each spouse in a marriage should experience a sense of need, want, acceptance, and selfless love. And knowing the fundamental distinctions between how men and women regard sex in general is one of the keys to establishing this kind of connection. Due to these disparities, men and women have different expectations of one another, which frequently causes confusion, annoyance, and disappointment. The following graph provides a comprehensive overview of the distinctions between men and women in this domain. This chart analyzes general tendencies and differences between men and women and how they regard sex, therefore it is clear that it is not an absolute comparison.

When I first got married, I had no idea that my husband and I had different sexual preferences. In addition to my ignorance, I had been misled by pornography, lies told in the locker room, and representations of sex in the media. It was a sexual issue waiting to happen in a public area. As a result, even though my husband and I were attracted to one another and had a fulfilling sexual relationship, there was a great lot of stress on both sides of the marriage due to misaligned sexual expectations. Years passed before we were able to respect our differences and finally understand them. Our sexual intimacy and pleasure grew considerably as we developed in these areas. We stopped having unreasonable expectations for one another or expecting one another to behave in a certain way beyond what our natures are.

Here are some of the key lessons we discovered that can assist you in developing a successful sexual relationship with your spouse.

A.) Women Are Emotionally Stimulated Whereas Men Are Stimulated Visually

Males are physically segregated.
While women's relationships, comprehensive emotional oneness, and security may be of larger importance, physical oneness, diversity, and sex are given high value. Although they are not completely emotionally deaf, women are significantly better able to respond to emotional input than men are. Men find it challenging to comprehend this. Due to this, many men neglect to communicate to their spouses and gently satisfy their romantic and emotional demands. Men pay a high price for this lack of emotional support in the realm of sex. Every man needs to understand that simply taking off his clothing won't make his wife feel more attracted to him sexually. Because their spouses pay attention to them and communicate to them throughout the day, women become more receptive. Beyond their emotional state, women rarely react to sex. This does not preclude a woman from giving

herself sexually to her husband,if she doesn't feel like it . It simply means that her sexuality and emotional temperament go hand in one. In order to comprehend why God created women in this way, we must comprehend that God is not just interested in sex but also in the total integrity of the relationship.

God therefore intended married sex to function to its full capacity only in the presence of genuine care and compassion. The antithesis of this is a typical scenario in which a self-centered husband neglects his wife until evening and then expects his emotionally deprived wife to engage in sexual activity. God, in His perfect wisdom, devised a mechanism that prevents jerks from enjoying excellent sex. Respecting our spouses' individual differences is the key to having the best sex possible. This means that a guy must provide for his wife in a compassionate and selfless way. Included in this is the crucial component of romance, which simply refers to a husband initiating actions that pursue and appease his wife on her level of need and want. When a husband behaves in this way, his wife opens up to him sexually and responds to him. The sexual nature of a man differs greatly. The visual nature of men is strong. It is an irrefutable fact, yet women may have trouble understanding it. A wife must be aware of the fact that her husband can be sexually aroused very rapidly just by looking at her in order to satisfy his needs.

Women often dismiss this problem and so frustrate their husband's demands because they are considerably more critical of their own bodies than men are, and because they do not respond visually as strongly as men do. Husbands want to view their wives' bare bodies, and women need to understand this. Although flannel nightgowns and pitch-black bedrooms are many women's sexual havens when they don't want to reveal themselves, they are the antithesis of a man's ability to experience sexual fulfillment. A lady must appreciate and satisfy her husband's visual demands just as a guy must comprehend and meet his wife's emotional needs. This entails stepping outside of her comfort zone to reveal her body to her husband both before and during sex while wearing lovely lingerie to please her spouse, she would expose her body to him before and during intercourse. You only need to look at how they sin to grasp the distinctions between men and women in the field of sex. Women flock to soap operas and romance novels to wrongly satisfy their emotional needs, while males turn to pornography to wrongly satisfy their visual needs. We must learn to value one other's uniqueness and provide for each other's wants rather than seeking fulfillment sinfully outside of our marriages.

B.) Men Need Sexual Touching, And Women Need Non-Sexual Affection

One of the most perplexing contrasts between men and women is this one. When we don't see this fundamental distinction between us, sex turns into a bittersweet struggle of wills. An aggressive husband roughhousing, grabbing his wife's genitals as she complains and assumes a sexually protective stance is a familiar scenario that is played out in numerous bedrooms. They both become frustrated as a result of having their wants ignored.

Men must comprehend that their wives require gentle, non-sexual contact throughout the day and during sex in order to feel pleased in sex. A lady has a strong craving for this. She experiences a sense of emotional worth and care from it. She gets more sexually responsive the more kind, non-sexual attention a man shows his wife. The way a man is built and thinks is the exact opposite of this. Because of this, the majority of men believe that physical contact with their spouses is the best way to get them to turn on. This is bad because it prevents sexual fulfillment and instead causes frustration. But, wives must realize that their husbands want to have direct sexual contact with them. It fulfills a deep need in a man and is incredibly gratifying and arousing for him. Consequently, when husbands and wives get along well and respect each other's unique personalities, their intimate moments will feature a loving husband gently caressing and touching his wife while she feels his penis and other sexually stimulating portions of his body.

Evidently, a woman needs direct stimulation to her clitoris in order to have an orgasm when the intensity of the sexual encounter increases. This can be done in a variety of ways, but it must be done tenderly in a way that meets her need and doesn't overlook her general need for gentle, non-sexual attention. A wife could also have other parts of her body, like her breasts, that she likes her husband to stroke and caress. It must be carried out in a way that appeals to her, though. Selfishness is the most hazardous factor that imperils sexual joy. Couples who reject their sexual differences guarantee that they will experience frustration and unhappiness together. The finest sex is had , when both partners participate and are making an effort to satisfy each other's wants. The couple that experiences sexual fulfillment in their marriage is made up of two sexually sensitive and altruistic individuals.

C.) Men And Women Have Different Levels Of Sexual Need And Achieve Orgasms Differently.

Most males are more sexually inclined than their wives. This indicates that they have a stronger desire for sex and think about it more frequently. This is especially true for younger men, between the ages of eighteen and forty-five. Women's desire for sex frequently grows as they get older. A portion of this is attributable to their spouses' increased emotional security. Also, women may become more open to having sexual relations if they are no longer afraid of getting pregnant or if they are more accepting of their sexuality. Men's sexual drive declines as they age as a result of their testosterone level gradually declining.

A man typically starts to notice this alteration in his forties or fifties. Hence, it is feasible for either spouse to desire sex more frequently or less frequently than the other throughout the course of a marriage. Their desires are rarely exactly the same. On average, men desire sex more than their wives, but I have given advice to numerous angry wives whose husbands showed no interest in having sex. All of this is being said primarily to demonstrate the importance of accepting one another despite the fact that we don't always experience the same level of sexual intensity or need at the same time. Being judged, disregarded, or treated unfairly as a wife or husband is distressing or having a partner reject your expression of a sexual yearning. We all have needs, so when we reject our spouse's needs, we are also rejecting them.

I'll never forget the young couple I gave advice to when they were about to break up. Their main issue was that she was irritated by his constant need for sex. I heard a typical young husband explaining his desire for sex with his wife as well as the rejection and embarrassment he felt from her as I listened to him explain his side of the tale. His wife said that she didn't accept his sexuality while I listened to her account of the events. She was completely prepared for him to have little sex needs. She rebuffed his attempts outright, calling him perverted for desiring so much sex, and accused him of being such. No matter how much rejection or shame a couple heaps on one another, sex is a fundamental desire, especially among men. A man and woman can share goodwill and closeness when this need is recognized and acknowledged. Serious issues and sexual angst arise when it is misinterpreted and rejected. Understanding how men and women experience orgasms is the next step in embracing how our sexual receptivity varies. To be fulfilled sexually, males must have orgasm. But women might still feel fulfilled having sex with their spouses without having an orgasm. Although most guys find this challenging to comprehend, it is true nonetheless. During sexual activity, men virtually always have orgasm while women very rarely do. It is challenging for a woman to have an orgasm during sex since her clitoris, which is outside of and above her vagina, is her major sexual organ and the one that generates orgasms. Thus, in order for a woman to experience orgasm, her clitoris must be stimulated. Although she can enjoy sex without having an orgasm, most women frequently yearn for them.

When a woman wants to experience an orgasm, she should let her husband know and give him instructions on how to appropriately stimulate her. A husband must take his time, be considerate, and pay attention to his wife in order to satisfy her need for an orgasm. Some men have an impulsive desire for sex and are simply concerned with satisfying their own desires. Their wives feel abused and sexually frustrated as a result. Guys need to realize that women acclimate to sex more gradually. To feel sexually satisfied, they need attention prior to, during, and after intercourse. Males have a near-instantaneous sexual arousal. Men may attempt to pressure their wives into giving a sexual reaction that they are unable to do without the prosper care.

No matter how men are sexually wired, they need to understand that their women are different and need to be given the right attention and care both before and during sex in order to be at their best. This does not imply that all marital sex must be experienced in the same manner. A "quickie" can occasionally be rewarding. This typically means that a partner is given access to a spouse's body, most frequently a wife, in order to satisfy an instant sexual demand. A "quickie" is just sex that is had quickly and spontaneously during an encounter or through some other method. A "quickie" won't usually be enough for a woman to have an orgasm and feel completely satisfied sexually. Women must be courted and cared for before sex.

A woman requires foreplay, love, loving dialogue, and pleasure inducing clitoral stimulation during sex. A woman can experience an orgasm and sexual satisfaction in this way. Men and women have very distinct sexual needs, as I've already mentioned. Sexual contentment results from acknowledging these variations and honoring our spouses' sexual preferences.

What percentage of the information you read in this chart applies to your own sexual interaction with your spouse? When we go through material like this, we are reminded of how God takes a man and a woman with such disparate needs and uses those disparities to enhance their compatibility and produce a relationship where they are "one body."

Most guys tend to concentrate on a relationship's physical features. The sight of their wife stimulates, draws, and captivates them. When they are stimulated physically or visually, they get instantly thrilled or at least interested. Most males may become physically intimate in a matter of minutes. Once sexual release occupies his primary thought, it dominates his attention. Guys are now prepared to begin the process of seeking sexual release through sexual activity. In general, men prioritize sex significantly more than women do, and women have a distinct orientation that necessitates a different strategy. Women are more focused on relationships. A woman seeks emotional oneness; a male seeks physical oneness. Men are stimulated by sight, smell, and their bodies. The lady is stimulated by touch, attitudes, acts, words, and the entire person. A man needs to be admired, respected, and physically required. The lady requires time to get used to the sexual act, as well as compassion, love, and emotional need. The sexual reaction of the guy is acyclical, or available anytime, wherever. The woman's reaction is cyclical, which means there are periods when she is more eager to engage in sexual activity than at other times. Whereas a woman is significantly slower, a guy responds sexually by getting thrilled quickly. A guy is focused during sexual activity, but a woman may be quickly distracted by thoughts of the kids, the doors, the sounds outside or insignificant events that are happening nearby. The release, orgasm, is the final significant difference. A male will typically have a rather brief, powerful, and physically demanding sexual release. A wife shouldn't be concerned about this because God made her spouse in this way. You see, this intensity wasn't intended to hinder a connection; rather, it was meant to build and enhance it. A husband's feeling of intimacy to his wife is one outcome of this potent sexual release. God has infused it into his very character, even though he does not explicitly state it. In a way that satisfies this most intimate need, he is pulled to his wife. When a husband concentrates on the body, it will lead to tension in the marriage when men overlook the fact that the woman needs the connection and instead emphasize the physical aspect of sex. Yet spouses frequently miss the important connection between a man's sexuality and his self-image. Because their men are such sexual beings, many wives say they feel offended. To a male, this approach conveys rejection. To just endure his advances, disregard his wants for sex, or refuse to initiate sex with him is to rip his self-esteem to shreds. We invite you to pray about your sexual connection as a couple. Pray that you all will be kind to one another. Pray God to give you the knowledge and courage to provide for one another. You can be led and guided to become a better lover by the Holy Spirit. The Holy Spirit wants to make me a better lover, you might ask. Absolutely! In the "afterglow" of sharing in love with your wife, I would strongly advise husbands to pray loudly for her. There is no better time than this to pray, "Dear Jesus, thank you for this woman you have given me. Thank you for what we just experienced together, for her, for her love, and for her confidence in me as a man. That has to provide your lady a sense of nourishment, esteem, and love because that is what this is all about.

You and your partner have learnt how to respond sexually. God wants you to experience this amazing act of oneness that He has prepared for marriage and to learn how to pleasure each other together. Even if you were unaware of the distinctions between men and women, and as a result, you went through some grief, God can and will restore this aspect of your marriage as you seek Him and live according to His truth. Decide to educate yourself about God's morals and sexual relationship-related laws.

<h1 style="text-align:center">SECTION 2</h1>

<h1 style="text-align:center">ELIMINATE THE COMMON ENEMIES OF SEXUAL FULFILLMENT</h1>

couples will encounter sexual fulfillment for a lifetime, they should appropriately answer a few normal issues that can undermine their expectations for progress. Despite the fact that these issues can be survived, they should be viewed in a serious way and tended to appropriately. Unfortunately, many couples who wed with extraordinary sexual energy and fascination between them wind up battling or in any event, separating, referring to their sexual issues as the essential issue. Since sexual issues are one of the fundamental explanations behind strain between wedded couples, I will address three shared adversaries of sexual satisfaction and how you can survive them.

A.) Unresolved Anger And Hurts.

Outrage is unavoidable in each marriage. It is basically impossible that two individuals can live together without ending up being angry at one another eventually. Indeed, even solid couples can encounter outrage consistently. This might astonish you, yet all the same it's valid. The issue isn't whether we will encounter outrage; the issue is the manner by which we manage it. I have guided many couples throughout the long term who experienced sexual issues. A lot of them were encountering sexual challenges because of unsettled outrage between them. There is a direct association between our feelings and our sexual reactions. At the point when we are resolving issues in our relationships effectively, our sexual experiences are unhindered as we express our actual love. Notwithstanding, when issues stay irritating and outrage assembles, our sexual cravings and reactions change. I accept unsettled outrage is the most risky component in marriage. It is basic for married couples to speak the truth about their feelings and to permit genuineness from one another. It is likewise fundamental for managing outrage rapidly. The Messenger Paul in Ephesians 4:26 advises us to concede our resentment yet not to allow the sun to go down on it. Sexual wellbeing isn't simply an issue of how our bodies answer sexual boosts. It is a lot of words upon our profound state. Unsettled outrage implies there are sensations of harm, doubt, or on the other hand infringement between us. The more these issues gather and stay unsettled, the more it will be reflected in our sexual reactions. Sex goes about as both a thermometer and an indoor regulator in a marriage. As an indoor regulator, sex improves marriage. Great sex really expands the close to home temperature of the marriage and assembles sensations of closeness and altruism. Notwithstanding, sex likewise goes about as a thermometer, and that implies it mirrors the condition of the relationship. Sexual issues might commonly at any point be expected to unsettled struggle. An absence of sound sexuality between a couple for any huge timeframe is an admonition signal that could be reflecting unsettled outrage. Damages and dismissals, particularly those from an earlier time, can likewise emphatically influence an individual's capacity to open up physically. Each individual comes into marriage with a specific level of close to home injuries from an earlier time, yet except if they are settled, a feeling of dread toward closeness can be the outcome. An individual who has been profoundly injured, either from a past marriage or relationship, frequently lives in a feeling of dread toward being dismissed or harmed once more. This dread can devastatingly affect their capacity to be physically open and responsive. Assuming you perceive any of these issues in your relationship, that's what I suggest you tell the truth and permit your companion frankly. Discuss your sentiments as you resolve to pardon your life partner and not to permit outrage and close to home injuries to remain. In the event that you can't determine an issue or issues among you and your mate, then, at that point, seek guidance from a Christian chief or expert. Your marriage is excessively essential to permit issues to remain unre-tackled. It denies you of the closeness and delight each wedded couple can and ought to encounter.

B). Deception.

The conviction that wrongdoing will improve sex or restore a slowed down sexual coexistence is a hazardous element for any marriage.
The world we live in is loaded up with sexual double dealing. We are encircled by it consistently, and if we don't watch out, it will taint our reasoning and damage our relationships. Today, men are being tricked by erotic entertainment. A man need not pass on his home to be defied day to day with sensual pictures from TV, maga-zines, PCs, and films. Little assuming any of the sexual symbolism around us is reliable with scriptural truth. Satan, in his longing to annihilate us, assaults us with his blazing rockets of trickery. Erotic entertainment is Satan's exceptional weapon to annihilate men and marriage. It isn't anything not exactly evil sex training. Porn depicts ladies as sex objects without profound necessities. Subsequently, as a man sees porn, he is persuaded to think that "ordinary" ladies need sex however much he does and in the very way he does. This definitely persuades him to think that something is off about his significant other and that he is being ransacked. I have seen

numerous men misuse and forsake their spouses as an immediate consequence of the trickiness of porn. The fact that leads us into makes us as men, we should understand that sexual entertainment clearly false duplicity and subjugation. The more sexual entertainment a man sees, the more he should see to fulfill the ever increasing craving it makes. Likewise, the more sexual entertainment a man sees, the raunchier it should be to fulfill him. More regrettable still, as a man raises his sexual entertainment compulsion, he will ultimately need to carry on the way things are playing out. He will frequently attempt to involve his significant other in his carrying on, which dehumanizes her and makes her nothing under an object of vaginal masturbation for him. Or on the other hand, more awful still, he will go external to his union with an attempt to encounter the existence envisioned in porn. God has planned sex to be fulfilling just when it incorporates closeness. Closeness implies an inward closeness and profundity of relationship that incorporates life elements. Consequently, sex in marriage is the main sex that can fulfill in light of the fact that it draws from our encounters in general and everyday issues together. Porn side steps each and every everyday issue and commitments sexual satisfaction exclusively on an actual level. This is the quintessence of the lie of erotic entertainment. I have known men who have annihilated their lives chasing after illegal sexual delight. They are headed to continually take care of the beast of sexual fervor, however with truly decreasing levels of fulfillment. Their destroyed lives are the final product of the trickery of erotic entertainment. Numerous ladies are additionally being misdirected connected with sex.

Romance books, dramas, films, Web discussion channels, sites, and female erotica all court a lady's varying sexual disposition. Once more, however we seldom see them in that capacity, they are types of sinister sex training. Allow me to involve romance books for instance. They are quite often composed by ladies and for ladies.

Romance books depict reality in a way inverse from male-situated sexual entertainment. They invigorate ladies by minimizing the sexual idea of men and over-emotionalizing them. Since they are composed of ladies and for ladies, they swing to the sexual viewpoint of ladies and overlook the truth of the sexual power of men.

The most terrible aftereffect of romance books and female erotica is that they persuade ladies that there are men out there (in contrast to their spouses) who are substantially more profound and considerably less sexual. The peril is that a tricked viewpoint is profoundly embedded in ladies that multiple occasions makes them judge and reject their spouses as they persuade themselves they are missing out on "genuine romance." As married couples, we should dismiss the lies of Satan and decline to be engaged or energized by them. As we do this, we should understand reality with regards to sex. It is just satisfying as we both turn our hearts to one another and strive to meet each other's varying requirements. We are made physically unique, and we make significant harm to our relationships when we reject those distinctions and attempt to adjust our life partners into our picture. This is precisely the exact thing sexual entertainment and female erotica do and why they are so perilous.

C.) Stress.

We as a whole realize we live in a high speed culture. The requests of occupations, youngsters, housework, financial pressures, and different issues can leave one or the two mates depleted and physically lethargic. This isn't an issue on the off chance that it happens rarely. Notwithstanding, when it happens routinely, it can cause profound disappointment for the life partner whose sexual necessities are being disregarded. The principal thing we should do to eliminate pressure from our lives is to focus on. Despite what certain individuals might think, you can't have everything. Life should be focused on to find true success, and each need should be shielded from contending requests. God made union with be the most noteworthy need in existence except for our own relationship with Him. He communicated this obviously in Genesis 2:24, where He expressed that a man would need to pass on his dad and mom to be joined to his significant other. This implies that the most elevated need throughout everyday life (the blood bond among ourselves and our folks) should turn into a lesser need for marriage. Taking stock of our lives is essential consistently, particularly when we are encountering pressure. As we do, we want to inspect those things that set expectations of us genuinely, emotionally, and intellectually.

Assuming we understand that the more prominent needs of our lives (God, marriage, youngsters) are being denied their legitimate spot by lesser things (companions, work, sports, leisure activities, amusement), we should be able to reprioritize or even eliminate the lesser things. I gave up golf for quite some time due to this very issue. I have consistently wanted to play golf, yet prior in our marriage, it was an icon. I would go straightforwardly from work to the fairway and afterward get back home depleted and reluctant to address her issues.

Be that as it may, I anticipated that she should serve me and meet my sexual requirements. She was profoundly angry, and it turned into a significant issue in our marriage. Surrendering golf was a penance for me, yet as I think back, it was worth it for the unbelievable closeness we have today. It doesn't make any difference how effective you are working or how much cash you have on the off chance that you're disturbed at home. Looking at this logically, you will concur that nothing in life can possibly make you as blissful or as hopeless as your marriage. Along these lines, it deserves the most elevated level of penance and speculation. Settle on a choice to focus on your marriage first and make anything that penances or changes are important to give your life partner the significant investment the individual merits. One more typical issue of pressure connects with kids and housework. For any spouse needing great sex, he should take on the obligation to assist with the children and the home. It is out of line for a man to get back home from work and sit before the TV anticipating that his significant other should bear the weight of kids and housework and afterward to come to bed depleted, however able to ener-getically address his issues. Whether or not a lady works at home or outside the home, a spouse needs to tell his better half that he is her accomplice in each everyday issue. A shrewd spouse who needs to appreciate great sex will bear the weight for his better half and permit her to have a period of rest and unwinding before sex. An impulsive spouse will overlook his better half and decline to acknowledge liability regarding the home, youngsters, funds, or other issues that cause her pressure. In managing the normal burdens of life, it is likewise really smart to design sex ahead of time. This positively doesn't forestall unconstrained sex; it simply implies making a unique date for sex on normal events so the two mates can get ready appropriately. At the point when our kids were youthful and we had many requests on us, this is the very thing that I did. We would choose ahead of time to have a night together and get it going. These were generally incredible times since we focused on and anticipated them. Likewise, every few months, we would go for an evening or two to an inn just to be distant from everyone else together. At the point when I look back on our marriage and how we prevailed in exceptionally active times, I accept this was a key explanation. Really we didn't allow conditions to direct us; we focused on being together and appreciating sex, and we got it going. Another issue connected with pressure: kids are under pressure like never before, and it straightforwardly influences us as guardians. Very much like grown-ups, numerous kids accept they must have all that and be all over the place. In the event that their requests and wants aren't observed by shrewd guardians, youngsters will grow up being passed through existence with their folks as the "escorts." Despite the fact that each parent should work and forfeit for their youngsters, sound judgment ought to let us know where to lay out legitimate boundaries. I know many couples whose connections have been harmed and, surprisingly, annihilated in view of the unreasonable requests of their youngsters. Keeping your kids' timetables reasonable will significantly diminish the pressure you experience as a couple and as a family.

SECTION 3

OVERCOME THE BARRIERS TO FULFILLING SEX

Notwithstanding the shared adversaries of sexual satisfaction, there are likewise a couple of obstructions that are significant for you to know how to survive. A portion of these boundaries can be unobtrusive in the manner they influence us, yet they are still factors that can adversely influence the level of sexual fulfillment we experience in marriage.

That is the reason I have included them here, alongside useful ways of managing them.

A.) Spiritual Barriers

As I referenced before, many individuals work in the conviction that sex is essential for Satan's domain and not God's. They have a misguided judgment that to truly appreciate sex, they need to get over into the domain of haziness that an individual can't be otherworldly and sexual simultaneously. I accept it's about time we salvage the subject of sex from Satan's camp and remember it as sacred in God's eyes. Having a profoundly otherworldly relationship with God doesn't reject a man or lady from having a profoundly sexual relationship with their life partner. Keep in mind, sex was God's thought in any case! His longing is for couples to appreciate sex to its fullest with next to no disgrace or culpability. Satan believes we should feel that God is a priss, yet truly He made sex for reproduction as well with respect to our pleasure. It is one of the best advantages of marriage. Rather than giving the fallen angel credit for something so brilliant, we want to say thanks to God for this wonderful gift.

B.) Physical Barriers

There are two perilous limits in our general public today connected with our bodies and sex. One limit is the drive for actual flawlessness, which makes many individuals take to undesirable drastic courses of action to attempt to make themselves more appealing. It additionally implies that more individuals are requesting unreasonable actual guidelines of their life partners. I as of late directed a couple who were isolated and very nearly separate. The spouse continually reprimanded his better half for her weight. Not exclusively were his guidelines unreasonable, yet he continually contrasted her and ladies' bodies he found in magazines and on TV. She felt dismissed and overpowered. Another limit is when individuals misuse their wellbeing regardless of what it means for their life partners and their sexual relationship. Whether it is weighty drinking, substance addiction, or stoutness, these issues straightforwardly influence our sexuality and our relationships. Subsequently, we should acknowledge liability to deal with ourselves. Practice and smart dieting propensities likewise influence sexuality. Individuals who work-out consistently have better cardiovascular abilities, which straightforwardly influence bloodstream to the private parts as well as different regions of the body. This results in more noteworthy responsiveness and sexual excitement. Certain prescriptions can likewise affect sexual execution. Antidepressants, pulse, and diabetic prescriptions can have secondary effects that adjust sex drive or capacity. As we age, chemical changes can likewise be an element. Diminished degrees of testosterone or estrogen can influence sex drive, and they can for the most part be dealt with successfully with drugs. Barrenness in men is another condition that requires clinical consideration. If you are encountering worry in any of these areas, don't put it off any more. Make a meeting with your primary care physician and get the assistance you require, for your own wellbeing and the strength of your marriage. Past the issue of wellbeing are the issues of cleanliness and prepping. A man ought to be certain that he is perfect and doesn't move toward his significant other with messy hands, and so forth. Likewise, managing nose hair and ear hair, having clean teeth and great breath, washing, utilizing cologne, being clean-cut, and it are all to dress well. Assuming we maintain that our spouses should be drawn to us and free themselves dependent upon us physically, we should comprehend that it is so critical to them that we care for ourselves. To our spouses, the manner in which we groom ourselves is a genuine proportion of the amount we care about them and the amount we will put into the relationship. For a lady, preparing implies that she really focuses on her hair, dress, and generally appearance.

I as of late saw a lady who was alluring and very much kept before she wedded, however promptly subsequently she "went to pieces." I see her and her better half routinely, and clearly she is taking him for granted. The standard she utilized for her appearance before their wedding dropped promptly subsequently. Despite the fact that her better half is outwardly invigorated, her negligence for her appearance is genuinely a dismissal for his requirements.

Unfortunate preparation and cleanliness are perilous fixings that establish a negative sexual climate. On the other hand, really focusing on our wellbeing and prepping adds a strong dynamic to a positive sexual air.

C.) Volitional Barriers

Some two or three arrive at a stalemate where one life partner is reluctant to address different issues.

Anything the reason might be, an absence of obligation to address each other's issues significantly affects the capacity to answer physically to one another. A fruitful marriage expects that both couples say, "I'm completely dedicated to this marriage in great times and in terrible times. I won't pull out or become self-satisfied. I will forcefully address your issues, anything that it takes." When a companion misses the mark on responsibility and on second thought shows an uncooperative or unfriendly demeanor, it typically requires looking for help through directing. Recall that seeking guidance is certainly not an indication of shortcoming; it is an indication of insight.

Your marriage is excessively critical to disregard such a difficult issue. Find an instructor who depends on God's Promise as the norm, and let him guide you to tracking down an answer.

SECTION 4

WORK TO CREATE AN ATMOSPHERE OF SEXUAL PLEASURE

When you comprehend the distinctions in your life partner and how to defeat the shared adversaries and hindrances to sexual satisfaction, you can seek after unhindered delight. This is one of the best gifts of life and marriage. We are sexual creatures, and point of fact, sex is the best actual delight throughout everyday life. As I said toward the start of this book, God made marriage in heaven referred to Eden, important as "joy and enjoyments." In doing as such, God obviously uncovered His plan and longing for marriage that it would be a position of sexual joy and joy. Indeed however basically every wedded couple participates in sex, only one out of every two or three encounters a similar level or recurrence of delight. Couples can enormously improve the level of sexual delight in their relationships by making a great air. The following are three fixings that make an air of sexual satisfaction and joy:

A.) Communicate Honestly And Openly About Your Sexual Needs And Desires

The main way we can really know how to satisfy our mates physically is for them to tell us. This can and ought to occur previously, during, and after sex. This kind of correspondence occurs as we both focus on sharing and on getting what is shared. We should make an air in which our life partners feel great sharing their sexual necessities and wants without being dismissed or censured. Clearly, if our companions share something with us that is wicked or abuses our still, small voice, we don't need to acknowledge it. Nonetheless, regardless of whether it is corrupt and abuses us, we should watch out for how we answer. We really want to tell our mates that we will in any case adore them and are focused on them physically. This is the kind of thing ladies manage a ton.

A few spouses believe their wives should accomplish something that disregards them. A lady must be consistent with her soul without harming the relationship with her significant other or conveying dismissal. Then again, numerous men become disappointed with their spouses since they just speak with them physically through negatives. At the end of the day, instead of straightforwardly sharing their longings and what satisfies them, spouses hold their sexual remarks for when the husband is doing something wrong. "Stop!" "Don't do that!" "That damage!" "I could do without that!" remarks like that are the main instruction a few men get to direct them in attempting to satisfy their spouses. This isn't as it were disappointing, yet it is additionally confounding and counterproductive. Pretty much every man I know needs to physically satisfy his better half. This doesn't imply that men don't have their own concerns. It simply implies that most men want to satisfy their spouses, however they rely upon positive guidance to succeed. This is particularly significant on the grounds that people are so divergent in their profound and actual plans and wants. A positive sexual climate should incorporate correspondence that makes an unmistakable guide that leads married couples to satisfy each other's sexual cravings.

Concerning this issue, there is another significant point that can block sound correspondence. Certain individuals, particularly ladies, are raised with harsh perspectives concerning sex. It is generally imparted through a parent's sexual remarks and perspectives. In the event that guardians view sex in a negative light, they will typically communicate this straightforwardly or in a roundabout way to their kids. The impacts can be significant upon a kid's future sexual relationship with a life partner. Once more, I need to underline the point that God made sex and it is lovely. God's ideal will is for you to have a pleasurable and invigorating sexual coexistence with your life partner. Try not to be embarrassed about sex or treat it as a no issue. Discuss your sexual cravings, and urge your mate to do likewise. Try not to allow Satan to deny you of the delight of sex by making it a messy subject. Sex is God's property, and it is quite possibly the best gift throughout everyday life. This is the appropriate method for figuring it out. Likewise, certain individuals view sex in a negative light due to a sexual sin or practice of their pasts. Assuming that you've accomplished something wrong, you really want to atone and accept God's pardoning. Be that as it may, don't let the slip-ups of your past hold you back from succeeding today. Sex, very much like anything more, can be fortunate or unfortunate. Utilize your past as a sign of what you shouldn't do. Allow God's Assertion to be your aide of what you ought to do. Assuming you're considering what the Good book needs to say regarding sexual joy, you can start by perusing the book of the "Tune of Solomon." Prepare to be astounded at how distinctively the Good book depicts sexual closeness in marriage. Likewise, many individuals, particularly ladies, have encountered sexual maltreatment from before. Now and again, this misuse was outrageous.

In the event that you don't carry your harmful past out from the shadows and permit the Master to mend you, your sexual wellbeing and marriage can be impacted in a negative manner. You genuinely must find support if essential and manage past maltreatment on the off chance that it is holding you back from opening yourself to sexual joy in marriage. There isn't anything that God can't recuperate or empower you to survive.

B.) Use Creativity And Energy In Giving Sexual Pleasure To Your Spouse.

Sex was made by God for two reasons. To start with, He believes we should multiply. Second, He believes we should encounter joy in marriage. As we seek after giving and getting joy in marriage, we want to go ahead and investigate the domains of sexual joy and to know where the limits are. As I've educated and mentored throughout the long term, I have had many individuals get some information about what is permitted and not permitted physically inside marriage. Much of the time, couples feel to some degree hesitant to explore different avenues regarding certain things since they dread they will sin or accomplish something wrong. Here are a portion of the normal things individuals get some information about:

- Oral sex
- Utilizing vibrators or sex toys
- Different sexual positions other than the preacher position
- Butt-centric sex
- Carrying on sexual dreams

In resolving these issues with couples, I first let them know that God believes them should appreciate sex. Likewise, I let them know that when something isn't explicitly taboo in Sacred writing, it by and large is on the grounds that it is permitted. A model is oral sex. I've heard a lot of ministers throughout the long term discuss how it is a transgression. In any case, there is no spot in Sacred text where it is prohibited. Similar rules apply to different practices recorded previously. In spite of the fact that I am not really supporting or suggesting them, I likewise don't accept an evangelist or any other person has the ethical position to let an individual know what the person should or shouldn't do in that frame of mind of the room on the off chance that the Book of scriptures hasn't taboo it. Here are the significant issues I accept you really want to think about in permitting or refusing any sexual practice:

Is it illegal in the Good book?

- Does it abuse my heart before God?
- Does it abuse my companion or is it against their will?
- Is this actually protected? Causes it to damage me or my life partner?
- Are there medical problems or dangers implied?

- Does this treat my life partner in a rude way or harm our relationship?

These are the significant inquiries to consider to assist you with finding a position of goal concerning your sexual boundaries. Once more, let me underscore that God believes you should have a great time and appreciate sex.

I accept there are wide boundaries for sexual satisfaction in marriage, and on the off chance that it feels far better to you and isn't against God's Promise, you ought to think about it. The best relationships are those where two individuals appreciate one another and encourage one another. You really must move toward sex according to this viewpoint and don't let the assessments of others direct your sexual practices. You understand better compared to anybody, with the exception of God, what you like and what is best for your marriage. When appropriately rehearsed, sex constructs and bonds your relationship and makes an environment of joy and pleasure. When you know how to determine questions connected with your sexual practices, focusing on satisfying your spouse is significant. Keep in mind, in the event that people could satisfy themselves physically, they wouldn't get hitched.

Couples rely on the inventiveness and energy of their mates to meet their sexual requirements. Regardless of whether they comprehend their mates' sexual requirements, esteeming them is significant. Likewise, ordinarily in marriage, one mate will actually want sex now and again when the other doesn't. The allurement is to decline their advances or to take part hesitantly. This can cause profound disappointment and hatred. Sexual satisfaction is capable when two individuals are delicate to each other and are focused on gathering each other's sexual requirements in an imaginative and fiery way. Never get sluggish or take your life partner for granted. Figure out what satisfies them, and figure out how to give sexual delight to your life partner. The more you put into it, the more your marriage will profit from your speculation.

C.) Find Positive Solutions To Sexual Problems.

There are times of marriage that carry with them extraordinary difficulties. A model is the point at which the ordinary oil of a lady's vagina during sex starts to evaporate as she enters her late thirties and early forties. Along these lines, she can start to encounter torment during sex. On the off chance that a response isn't found, a lady can start to oppose the lewd gestures of her significant other and really fear sex. The response to the issue is for a spouse to utilize KY Jelly or another water-based grease during intercourse or while straightforwardly invigorating his better half's clitoris. It replaces a lady's regular grease and reestablishes the joy of sex without torment. Likewise, as a man ages, he can experience issues accomplishing erections. As referenced before, this is clearly a difficult issue that requires an answer. With all of the clinical assistance accessible today, I recommend you look for the direction of a very much regarded doctor. There is no requirement for sexual brokenness to hold any man back from accomplishing erections and experiencing great sex until the end of his life. There are different issues that can adversely influence our sexual experiences, like the feeling of dread toward pregnancy, menopause, difficult disease, or the departure of a friend or family member. Despite what challenge we are confronting, we should confront it together and track down an answer. Particularly when a clinical issue is involved, we really want to counsel a doctor. At the point when the issues are close to home or otherworldly in nature, we want to get the assistance expected to keep our marriage as solid as could be expected.

We should recall that in any event, when we are confronting a difficult time throughout everyday life, our sexual requirements and our companions' necessities aren't guaranteed to disappear. In a sound marriage, sex is a consistent current that back and forth movements through our lives. Any time it stops for a critical time frame and under any condition, it should be managed as a difficult issue that requires consideration. Sound relationships are set apart by a disposition of sexual awareness and understanding. Each test or issue is met with a disposition of common concern and obligation to do what is best for the marriage.

SECTION 5

DO YOUR PART TO KEEP THE ROMANCE ALIVE

A book about sexual satisfaction couldn't be finished without including the subject of sentiment. At the point when the subject of sentiment comes up, there can be a ton of disarray since sentiment implies various things to various individuals. Ladies might consider a candlelight supper with significant discussion, while men might consider an interesting sexual experience. The significance of sentiment in marriage can't be undervalued.

Sentiment keeps your rela-tionship developing and your interests alive; without it there is a crumbling of the relationship. To assist you with understanding how to integrate sentiment into your marriage consistently, the following are three significant components to consider:

A.) Self-Started Pursuit.

At the point when you work on something for your companion that is startling and an unexpected treat, it imparts that the person is in your heart and that you truly care. For a spouse, it could mean preparation and setting up a unique feast for your better half. For a spouse it could mean sending her roses or a heartfelt card. Significantly, without being bothered or reminded, you put forth the attempt to seek after your companion in a vivacious manner.

B.) Creative Communication Of Value.

Perhaps the best thing you can do in marriage is to develop each other's confidence. Through heartfelt motions, you show your companion how significant the person is a major part of your life. Perhaps the most effective way to do this is to adulate your life partner to give verbal insistence. One more method for conveying esteem is through great habits being benevolent and deferential to one another. Many individuals treat outsiders better than they treat their mates. In a solid marriage, it's vital that you are obligated to one another's sentiments and take care to show that you respect one another.

C.) Speaking Affection In Your Life Partner's Language.

People's significant necessities are altogether different, and you must comprehend these distinctions to be heartfelt on one another's conditions. A man's four essential necessities are honor, sex, fellow cooperation, and homegrown help. A lady's four fundamental requirements are security, transparent correspondence, non-sexual friendship, and administration. At the point when a spouse carves out an opportunity to have significant discussions with his better half consistently, it meets perhaps of her most prominent need. In spite of the fact that it's not one of his needs, it's a significant way for him to show his affection in her language. It's the equivalent when a spouse resolves to respect her better half and meet his sexual necessities, despite the fact that they're not equivalent to hers.

To lay it out plainly, sentiment makes a relationship extraordinary in light of the fact that two mates will forfeit to address each other's issues. They will exhaust investment to seek after one another in imaginative ways, and they do it because of a willing heart and merry demeanor. The best sentiment on the planet is when the two companions are meeting each other at their place of need. They aren't underestimating one another, and they haven't developed apathetic in their relationship. At the point when a spouse centers around tracking down better approaches to convey how significant his better half is to God and to him their marriage is in paradise. It's the equivalent when a spouse zeros in her energies and consideration on her significant other. At the point when the flash of sentiment is lighted in a marriage, the force of sexual satisfaction can improve. I trust this book has assisted you with figuring out the significant subject of sexual satisfaction in marriage. I supplicate you will actually want to prevail in encountering the best level of sexual delight and satisfaction in your marriage. God favors you.

CONCLUSION

This book helps in further developing couple conjugal fulfillment by featuring the requirement for consciousness of sexual quality. We should recall that sex is God's creation and that His craving is for us to appreciate it to its fullest inside the boundaries of marriage.